"Elyse Resch has taught me that the key to body positi
or strict rules, but about being in tune with your body
idea that we have to listen to our bodies and nourish o
on an individual basis. This book has been such a great tool for me, and I hope
who struggle with body issues are able to access this journal and use it to overcome their own
challenges."

> —Demi Lovato, recording artist, actress, and activist

"This journal is an emotional and practical tool kit—full of compassionate, reflective prompts for
healing and rediscovering joy and satisfaction from food. Wherever you may be on your journey,
this book opens the door to accessing deeply meaningful and transformative steps to take. It's the
book we've been waiting for; one that meets you at the intersection of wanting to change, and not
knowing how."

> —Sumner Brooks, MPH, RDN, CEDRD, coauthor of *How to Raise an Intuitive Eater*

"*The Intuitive Eating Journal* is a confidential, sometimes surprising conversation with a
fascinating person you don't know very well—your inner intuitive eater. And once you realize how
much the two of you have in common, it's like a delicious dish prepared by someone who knows
all about you and loves you anyway: both deeply nourishing and intensely soul-satisfying."

> —Jessica Setnick, MS, RD, CEDRD-S, creator of Eating Disorders Boot Camp, and
> author of *The Sleepless Dietitian's Big Book of Answers*

"In this sophisticated journal, Elyse Resch offers practical, compassionate, emotionally attuned,
and responsive prompts that are relevant for individuals of all ages—and body shapes and sizes—
to improve their relationship with themselves and with food. Drawing from her extraordinary
expertise, she engages the reader beautifully, helping them leave behind diet culture and honor
their emotions, needs, and bodies. I will be using this vital resource in my practice. It's brilliant!"

> —Jennifer L. Gaudiani, MD, CEDS-S, FAED, founder and medical director of the
> Gaudiani Clinic, and author of *Sick Enough*

"Elyse Resch's *The Intuitive Eating Journal* is a wonderful addition to your Intuitive Eating
toolbox. No matter where you are on your journey, this tool will help you cultivate a healthy
relationship with food, mind, and body. Say goodbye to diet culture once and for all."

> —Evelyn Tribole, MS, RDN, coauthor *Intuitive Eating,* and author of *Intuitive Eating
> for Every Day*

"Anyone who struggles in their relationship with food will find wisdom in these pages to help them heal. With thought-provoking questions and helpful explanations of key concepts, *The Intuitive Eating Journal* will resonate with readers of the other Intuitive Eating books, as well as those who are new to Intuitive Eating."

—Christy Harrison, MPH, RD, registered dietitian, and author of *Anti-Diet*

"Connect to yourself like never before with *The Intuitive Eating Journal*. Resch's thoughtful, reflective prompts will help you slow down and notice more from your experiences. You end up realizing that your own words offer the valuable wisdom you need to help you heal your relationship to food."

—Rebecca Scritchfield, RDN, author of *Body Kindness*

"A verifiable treasure trove of tools to build a joyful, peaceful relationship with food and cultivate respect for your body. Elyse freed me from the chains of diet culture four years ago, and I wish I had *The Intuitive Eating Journal* when I was first starting out. The prompts and exercises make you think, reevaluate, and redefine your relationship with food and movement on your own terms. Interesting, transformative, and liberating work!"

—Jessica Knoll, *New York Times* bestselling author of *Luckiest Girl Alive*

"Studies show that Intuitive Eating is linked to enhanced health and well-being—simply put, Intuitive Eating nurtures our bodies. The *Intuitive Eating Journal* represents a unique opportunity to dive deeply into each of the ten Intuitive Eating principles. The carefully crafted reflections prime us to explore personal experiences that have helped or hindered our Intuitive Eating journeys, and articulate ways we can continue to make peace with food and our bodies—wherever we are in our process."

—Tracy Tylka, PhD, professor of psychology at The Ohio State University, editor in chief of *Body Image*, and coauthor of *Positive Body Image Workbook*

THE

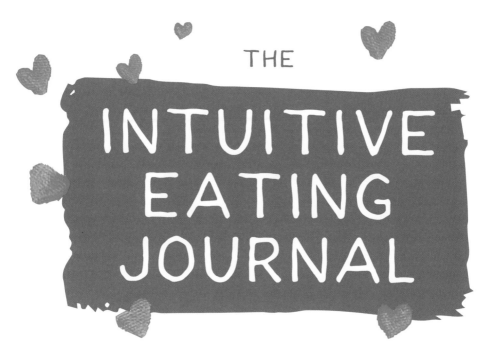

INTUITIVE EATING JOURNAL

Your Guided Journey for Nourishing
a Healthy Relationship with Food

ELYSE RESCH, MS, RDN

New Harbinger Publications, Inc.

Publisher's Note

Distributed in Canada by Raincoast Books

Copyright © 2021 by Elyse Resch
New Harbinger Publications, Inc.
5674 Shattuck Avenue
Oakland, CA 94609
www.newharbinger.com

Cover and interior design by Amy Shoup

Acquired by Ryan Buresh

Library of Congress Cataloging-in-Publication Data on file

Printed in China

23   22   21

10   9   8   7   6   5   4   3   2   1   First Printing

CONTENTS

INTRODUCTION

Intuitive Eating, the program on which this guided journal is based, starts from one truth:

We all come into this world with the wisdom to know how to eat.

Babies don't have theories and plans and rules about eating. They simply know when they are hungry and when they are full, and they act accordingly. But eating gets a lot more complex as we grow up. Most of us will encounter judgments about food, eating, and our bodies, and many of us internalize these judgments and listen to them instead of listening to our own innate wisdom. Diet culture weaponizes these judgments, privileges thin bodies, and teaches us to strive for an ideal weight which is usually unrealistic. It has distracted many of us from trusting our inborn intuitive wisdom so much that we don't even remember or believe that we have it.

But we do! The second truth Intuitive Eating holds is that *this wisdom never leaves us*. Even if you don't see it or trust it, it's there. This journal will help guide you through the noise of diet culture to a joyful, relaxed, and positive relationship with food and your body. Because all bodies deserve dignity and care.

Diets can cause us harm and pain. They are often abusive and can cause damage to many areas of our lives. For example, when we fail at a diet, we might stop engaging in activities that we enjoy and that offer us a better chance of achieving wellbeing. Diets and diet culture also promote weight stigma, which Intuitive Eating is committed to fighting.

AND—the kicker—diets simply don't work. They try to control you by depriving you of the foods you love and of a sufficient amount of them to feel satisfied. This backfires! Eventually, you'll burst out from this deep deprivation with an intense craving for everything you've given up, while at the same time, your healthy ego will rebel against this external control.

Intuitive Eating reassures you that only *you* know what is right for you. You can learn to listen to and trust your body's inborn wisdom. You are the expert!

ABOUT THIS GUIDED JOURNAL

This journal is a companion to your exploration of Intuitive Eating, and you can use it whether you know a lot about Intuitive Eating or nothing at all. My wish for this journal is to make Intuitive Eating about YOU. It will take you on a journey back to trusting the signals your body offers you. It will give you the space to set intentions and explore your thoughts and feelings about each of the ten Intuitive Eating principles.

My hope is that with this journal you practice being thoughtful and creative as you set your intentions and then as you discover the particular challenges you face along the way. With each prompt, you'll have space to note the actions you've taken or intend to take, and then to sit with the feelings that arise. Sometimes you'll be prompted to circle back to a previous experiment or to go a little deeper into what you're learning. For some prompts, you may want to use extra paper to further explore your thoughts and feelings—go for it.

You can use this journal front to back, or if you find that a chapter jumps out at you, by all means, begin there. You may find, however, that beginning with chapter 1, *Reject the Diet Mentality,* will give you the insight and motivation to fuel your journey.

The more time you spend on each principle, the more you'll become aware of your inner signals that form the foundation for your relationship with food and your body. The golden prize that you're striving for is the freedom that comes with knowing *you can trust your body to guide you through your eating world.* As you explore the principles of Intuitive Eating, this deep trust and freedom will help you let go of any fears and judgments you may have about letting yourself eat what you enjoy and will help you experience the great pleasure and satisfaction that eating can offer.

CHAPTER 1

Reject the Diet Mentality

Diet culture can trap you in a world of judgment. You feel bad for what you eat, how much you eat, and when you eat. You feel bad for being in the body you were born to be in. You feel that you need to change your body in order to be lovable or even acceptable. Diet culture can trick you into believing that your health is dependent on being small, or muscular, or some "approved" body shape that is somehow never quite *your* body's shape.

This chapter is designed to help you explore how having a "diet mentality" has affected you. Remember to be kind to yourself and to come from a place of curiosity, not judgment, when you revisit your diet history. You've done your best with the knowledge and resources you've had.

What might it be like to say "NO" to diet culture forever and open the door to a life of joy, satisfaction, and appreciation of your here-and-now body?

Let's find out!

Write about when you began your first diet—your introduction to diet culture. As best you can, recall your intentions—why did you start? What did you do to start, and what actions did you take to stay on the diet? What were the challenges? What feelings arose while you were on the diet? Write it all down and use extra paper if you run out of room. Be gentle with your former self.

💜 GO DEEPER: Do this exercise for more of your diet stories. What do you notice about the plans, hopes, thoughts, and feelings you've had while trying various diets? Are there any patterns?

What was your relationship with food like after you fell off your first diet? Were you driven to eat whatever you wanted, and as much as you could, to make up for what the diet restricted? Did you want to find another diet to try?

As best you can, describe your thoughts and feelings:

- about the diet experience.
- about not being on it anymore.
- about your body.
- about food.

Go back to the previous prompt and read what you wrote about how you felt after your first diet failed. Is this how you've felt after subsequent diets?

With your story fresh in your mind, imagine what it might be like to quit diet culture. What if you never go on another diet again?

Write a specific intention for breaking free from diet culture.

For example: "I intend to notice social media posts I see this week about the 'latest, greatest diet'. I will notice and write down my thoughts and feelings and then do *nothing about them*."

What might make it difficult to carry out your intention and how might you combat these challenges?

For example, your social media feeds may bombard you with diet culture messages, so you might unfollow or unsubscribe from some accounts.

Try it for a day, or a week, then reflect: How hard was it to keep your intention? What feelings did you have? What did you learn?

Think of as many actions as you can that will help you reject dieting. Here are some ideas:

O Stop weighing myself

O Throw out (or smash!) my scale

O Unsubscribe from diet media feeds

O Follow body liberation and Intuitive Eating feeds

O THROW AWAY my diet books

O Stop weighing and measuring food

What else?

O _____

O _____

O _____

O _____

O _____

O _____

O _____

O _____

O _____

O _____

Imagine you are finally free of diet culture. What is your relationship with food like? What's great about it? What's hard? What's confusing?

Starting with what you know so far about yourself, diet culture, and how diet culture differs from Intuitive Eating, what changes do you need to make in your life in order to do this work? These changes may have to do with the friends in your life, your family, your habits, or something else. How might you make these changes? What intentions could you set to help you? Write down whatever changes come to mind along with how you might accomplish them.

Come back to
this prompt from time
to time as you develop your
Intuitive Eating skills, habits, and
mindset. You can use what you
learn to keep improving your
relationship with food and
your body!

Are there any other intentions you'd like to set at this beginning of your journey toward Intuitive Eating? Write them here!

O _____

O _____

O _____

O _____

O _____

O _____

O _____

O _____

CHAPTER 2

Finding Satisfaction

Have you lost touch with the pleasure and delight you received from eating before you became trapped in diet culture? Watch the awe and excitement that come over a toddler's face the first time they taste ice cream, and you'll see what I mean. Imagine how wonderful it would be if eating became a great joy in your life (maybe for the first time in a very long time) and each meal brought you true satisfaction.

In this chapter, you'll begin reconnecting with *satisfaction*, which is at the core of Intuitive Eating. Satisfaction involves all your senses and how attuned to them you can be under various circumstances. It means savoring your food and allowing yourself the deep joy that comes with eating what truly pleases you.

Each of the ten principles is informed by finding satisfaction and getting the most satisfaction you can when you eat. This chapter will help get you there. Read through each exercise before you begin so you can plan how best to focus your attention to learn what each sense can offer you.

Begin to explore the different **tastes** of food.

Tastes you can try:

- ○ salty (like a pretzel)
- ○ sweet (like a cookie)
- ○ sour (like plain yogurt)
- ○ bitter (like a radish)
- ○ something called umami or savoriness (like hamburger)

Choose a taste to explore today and write it down. What's your plan to make this experience happen?

Afterward, write about what it was like. What thoughts, memories, or feelings did you have? Did you enjoy it? Would you like to try it again?

GO DEEPER: Try this exercise with each of the other tastes mentioned above. Write about your experience.

Begin to explore the different **textures** of food.

Textures you can try:

O silky smooth (like an avocado or tofu)

O crunchy (like a cracker)

O chewy (like a bagel)

O soft (like soft-serve ice cream)

O creamy (like full-fat yogurt)

O What else? _____

Which texture will you explore today? Write it down here, along with your plan for having this experience.

Afterward, write about what that was like. What thoughts, memories, or feelings did you have? Did the texture add to your satisfaction?

_____

_____

_____

_____

_____

_____

_____

_____

_____

_____

_____

_____

♥ GO DEEPER: *Mouthfeel* is the word for the physical sensations that food creates in your mouth. The mouthfeel and texture of your food can affect how satisfying it is. The textures you prefer can change from meal to meal, or day to day. Continue to experiment with different textures and pay attention to their impact on your satisfaction.

Begin to explore the different **aromas** of food. Does the smell of freshly baked cinnamon rolls make your mouth water? What about overcooked broccoli versus steaming-hot chicken soup?

Today, take time during one of your meals to consider the effect different aromas have on your appetite and your satisfaction level.

Write about the foods you ate and the aromas you encountered. Was it a positive, neutral, or negative experience? Did it bring up any memories, thoughts, or feelings? Reflect on how the aromas may have added to (or taken away from) your level of satisfaction.

Begin exploring the **appearance** of food. Is the food glistening from the oil used to prepare it? Does the crust look under-baked or perfectly toasted? Does the color assure you that the food is fresh? The visual appeal of food can enliven your anticipation of satisfaction from your meal. In fact, sometimes people get more satisfaction eating in a restaurant than at home, in part because being served a colorful or attractively presented meal is pleasing and comforting. The food just looks good!

Write about a meal you remember, where you think the appearance of the food (rather than its taste, texture, or aroma) was a big part of your satisfaction.

Now write about a meal where the appearance of the food took away from your feelings of satisfaction.

💜 GO DEEPER: Write some ideas for how you could make the appearance of your meals more interesting. Would a pretty plate, a fresh garnish, or a flower on the table increase your satisfaction? Experiment with making your meals more visually appealing. Write about what you discover.

Begin exploring the **temperature** of food. Do you like hot soup on a cold stormy day? Or maybe you always like your cold drinks with ice and your hot drinks piping hot, but your apple pie is more appealing at room temperature. Everyone's preferences are a little bit different!

What are your thoughts, memories, or feelings about the temperature of food and how temperature makes food satisfying or not? What are you discovering about your unique connection to food and drink temperatures?

Now let's begin to explore how to listen to other bodily sensations. Think about how some foods or meals make you feel content and satisfied, while others make you feel sleepy, or give you indigestion or a headache, even if they taste great. This is called **body feel.**

Choose a meal and when you're done eating, write about how you feel. Are you energized or drowsy? Are you physically satisfied? How about emotionally? Has this meal given you pleasure? Does the time of day matter? For example, if you eat pasta at lunch and feel drowsy, does it affect your day, or if you eat it at dinner, does the sleepy feeling add to its satisfaction? Write about your experience.

Try this
exercise again with
other foods and meals
to fully appreciate how
body feel affects
satisfaction.

Have you ever noticed that sometimes you get super hungry not long after eating, and other times you don't think about food for hours after a meal? The **staying power** of your food might make the difference in your satisfaction level.

Set an intention to notice the staying power of your breakfast. How long does a balanced breakfast like eggs, avocado toast, and fruit hold you before you get hungry again? Does your breakfast make you feel too full or does it keep you physically and emotionally satisfied for several hours?

How satisfied do you feel if you just eat a piece of fruit or a pastry in the morning? Even if you experience taste satisfaction, do you find that your body satisfaction lasts long enough for you? Write about your experience.

Begin to explore ways your **environment** affects how satisfied you feel after a meal. Here are some environmental factors to consider:

- How quickly or slowly you eat
- Distraction from the food (like the phone, TV, or computer)
- Chaos or conflict with other people during the meal
- Where you eat (home, restaurant, or car)
- What else?

This week, try eating slower or faster; while distracted or staying present; in different locations; alone or with friends or family.

Each time you do this, write about what you noticed. What effect did each environmental factor have on your feelings of satisfaction?

DAY ONE

DAY TWO

DAY THREE

38

DAY FOUR

DAY FIVE

DAY SIX

DAY SEVEN

Now explore how various **feelings** and **emotions** might affect your eating satisfaction. (There's a whole chapter about feelings coming up, but this is a helpful place to start exploring your relationship with food and your emotions.)

Start by writing a bit about what emotional states you think might take your appetite away and your satisfaction along with it. Write about which emotions might intensify the pleasure you get from eating.

Over the next few days, pay attention to your emotional state at mealtimes and your feelings of satisfaction from the meal. Write about what you notice.

CHAPTER 3

Honor Your Hunger

We've all felt hunger. Whether it's a baby screaming for food because hunger is likely a painful feeling, an adult going too long without eating and feeling intense pangs in the stomach, or the beginning of mild, subtle hunger—our bodies speak to us about our need to eat. As an Intuitive Eater, you learn to listen to your hunger signals, nourish your body, and feel the satisfaction that eating can bring you.

In this chapter, you will work on fine-tuning your hunger awareness and exploring the different kinds of hunger, including physiological hunger, taste hunger, emotional hunger, and others.

It's important to note that Honoring Your Hunger is simply a guideline. Be careful not to interpret Intuitive Eating rigidly or think that it means eating only when you're at the "perfect" hunger level and stopping at the "perfect" fullness level. This couldn't be further from the truth.

Start to explore the hunger signals that tell you when you're hungry and need to eat. Perhaps you don't notice hunger until you're ravenous, your energy is collapsing, and you feel a gnawing pain in your stomach. (At that point, you're experiencing something called *primal hunger.*) Or maybe you're able to detect the slightest inkling of hunger, a flutter in your stomach, a shift in your energy level, or another signal.

Here are some ways that people experience hunger:

- A slight sensation in the throat or esophagus
- A flutter in the stomach
- A gnawing in the stomach
- Stomach rumbling or growling
- Stomach pain
- Inability to focus or concentrate
- Light-headedness
- Tiredness
- Headache
- Moodiness

Over the next few days, notice which hunger signals are uniquely yours. When you notice a hunger signal, note the circumstances you were in and whether anything contributed to you being in touch with this signal. For example, perhaps it's quiet in the morning after you have just woken up and notice that you're hungry, or maybe you've been occupied all day, not noticing your body's signals, and hunger surges in with a force. Is the signal you feel pleasant, neutral, or uncomfortable?

Now that you've explored any hunger signals that you routinely feel, let's focus on levels of hunger. The Intuitive Eating hunger scale will help you identify what hunger number you're at, based on your physical sensations.

FEELINGS OF HUNGER & FULLNESS

Over Hungry	0	Painfully hungry. This is *primal hunger*. It's very intense and can actually hurt.
	1	Ravenous and irritable. An urgent need to eat.
	2	Extremely hungry. Immediate need to find some food.
Comfortable Eating Range	3	Fully hungry and ready to eat.
	4	Mildly hungry, begin noticing hunger.
	5	Neutral. Neither hungry nor full.
	6	Starting to feel satisfied.
	7	Comfortable fullness, feeling completely satisfied and content—a sign to stop.
Over Full	8	Beginning to feel a little too full. Beyond physically needing food.
	9	Extremely full and uncomfortable—everything feels tight.
	10	Stuffed and in pain. Maybe even nauseous.

For the next week, notice your hunger when you get up in the morning and answer each of these questions (using extra paper if you run out of room).

- What physical feelings did you notice?
- Rate these feelings on the hunger level chart.

- Are you extremely hungry, not at all, or somewhere in the middle?
- If you're not hungry (and you don't eat), when does mild hunger arise and what does it feel like? Do you eat at this point or put it off until lunch?
- If you sit down to eat breakfast, what is your hunger level?
- If you wait to eat until later, what is your hunger signal and hunger level when you finally eat? How many hours has it been since you got up?

DAY ONE

DAY TWO

DAY THREE

DAY FOUR

DAY FIVE

DAY SIX

DAY SEVEN

💜 GO DEEPER: If you discover you're not experiencing hunger in the morning, consider what may be blocking you from this feeling. Possibilities include eating late the night before, filling up with coffee, starting work and ignoring hunger signals. What else comes to mind?

If you are hungry but choose to ignore the signals, how does it impact your level of hunger and eating when you finally decide to eat? Notice this over a period of a couple days.

Today, set an intention to focus on how your hunger levels affect your satisfaction in the meal. Before each meal try to notice if you are comfortably hungry, ravenously hungry, or eating even though you're not hungry.

Explore your physical feelings when you eat. How does your hunger level before your meal impact how satisfying your food tastes, how much you eat, and how satisfied you are after finishing your meal?

If your exploration in this chapter has shown you that your eating is somehow out of touch with your hunger signals, how can you best stay tuned in to those signals?

Here are some ideas:

Practice letting go of dieting behavior. What dieting behaviors are keeping you from noticing your hunger signals? For example, do you have a habit of filling yourself up with liquids or air foods to avoid feeling hungry?

Reduce chaos in the morning. Try setting the alarm fifteen minutes earlier in the morning. Maybe it's best to eat after the kids have gone to school or to go out for breakfast occasionally if you can afford it.

Practice staying present to your hunger. Throughout the day, keep bringing your attention back to your body's hunger signals, as well as energy and mood signals.

What else? Write your own strategy.

Choose a tune-in strategy and try it for a few days. Write about what's hard, what's surprising, and what seems to help you tune in.

GO DEEPER: As you work through the factors that affect your ability to tune in to your hunger feelings, explore the emotions that come up for you while evaluating your habits.

As you know, it's possible to have an appetite for something even when you're not hungry. We call it **taste hunger** (as opposed to physical hunger which we've been exploring so far) and Intuitive Eating is just fine with it. Our brains have the capacity for all kinds of thoughts and feelings aside from the need for survival! (Remember, Intuitive Eating does not have rules—it simply gives you guidelines to experience more pleasure and satisfaction in your eating life.)

For today, notice the moments when you just want to eat something but aren't hungry. Write about that. Here are some questions to consider: What was the situation? What was the food? What are your usual thoughts and feelings about that food, and what were your thoughts and feelings about eating it today? Did you eat it? If not, why not? If you did, what thoughts and feelings did you have? Just notice everything: it is all useful information!

GO DEEPER: Write about your taste hunger experiences over a period of days. This will help you get used to noticing it and gather a bunch of information from your thoughts and feelings about your taste hunger.

After you spend some time getting to know your hunger, if you find that most of your eating is for taste hunger rather than physical hunger, write about that. What does this say to you about your relationship with food?

Do you ever find that you're eating because you want to soothe an emotion or push away a feeling? This is called **emotional hunger.** Food can be comforting! Don't judge yourself if you seek comfort in food, but take the opportunity to notice what's going on.

For a day or two, set an intention to notice when you seek food in connection with emotions. Write about what you find. What was the situation, including people, place, and time? What were your feelings before, during, and after this moment of emotional hunger, whether you ate the food or not? (This is just your first opportunity to think about emotional hunger! There is a whole chapter on this coming up.)

Have you noticed any other times or situations in which you want to eat even if you're not hungry? You've explored physical hunger, taste hunger, and emotional hunger. Now, spend a day focused on whether you can sense any other triggers for eating.

Possibilities include:

- *Energy-seeking hunger.* Feeling drowsy or low-energy leads you to think food could help.
- *Experience-sharing hunger.* Wanting to share the experience of eating with someone, even if you don't feel hungry.
- *Practical hunger.* Deciding to eat even if you're not hungry because you know you won't have the opportunity to eat later.

At the end of the day, write about any time you ate but weren't hungry. Describe the situation and how you felt. What worked for you? What didn't? Were you able to derive satisfaction when you ate but weren't hungry? This is the key to helping you balance eating for physical hunger versus any other reason.

If you didn't experience any of these other triggers for eating, what might you do if one came up?

♥ GO DEEPER: At this point on your journey toward Intuitive Eating, think deeply about your willingness to shed diet culture rules that tell you to eat only at some "exact" hunger level. Write about any rigid rules you've loosened up. If you are still holding onto some rules, write about any fears you have about letting them go. Remember to have self-compassion; making a significant change in your life can sometimes be difficult.

CHAPTER 4

Make Peace with Food

Making peace with food is one of the pivotal principles of Intuitive Eating. When you make peace with food, all foods are *emotionally* equivalent even if they are not *nutritionally* equivalent. This means you have the same emotional reaction whether you eat broccoli or a candy bar. You don't feel "good" for eating the broccoli or "bad" for eating the candy bar.

To feel truly at peace, and truly safe, you must trust that you will always give yourself permission to eat what you like. (Of course, practically, you can't always have access to the perfect food that satisfies all of your senses, but the key is to give yourself permission to enjoy what you like).

When you first begin to practice this principle, it may feel scary to allow yourself to eat exactly what you like. You might fear that you'll never stop eating some yummy food you've chosen. Rest assured that when you fully embrace this principle, your fears will dissolve.

We'll start by exploring two important forces: *deprivation* and *habituation*.

Any time something is forbidden to us, it triggers that itch inside us to get what we can't have. That itch is our *sense of deprivation,* and it's human nature. We are all driven by our unmet needs.

What triggers a feeling of deprivation in you? Is it a longing for more free time, sleep, or companionship? Are there foods you wish you could eat but think you shouldn't? When your sense of deprivation gets triggered, what does it feel like to you?

In the past, you may have felt deprived while dieting. You may have felt guilty if you ate a forbidden food, so as a result you would once again forbid it. During periods of deprivation, your feelings of guilt about eating the "wrong food" may have diminished. In diet culture, deprivation and guilt often work like a see saw—one goes up when the other goes down.

Diets tend to keep the see-saw moving. When you're being "good," deprivation feelings go way up, and you eventually eat something "forbidden." Then, deprivation sinks and guilt shoots up. Up and down, just like the seesaw (but much, much less fun).

Think about a time when you were restricting certain foods and found yourself on a deprivation/guilt seesaw. Write about that experience, including any feelings of guilt (and possibly shame) involved.

GO DEEPER: Write about any ways your feelings of guilt or shame may be receding as you become an Intuitive Eater and your deprivation lessens. Come back to this exercise after you finish this chapter and reflect on any changes.

When we feel secure that we have what we need and we'll always have as much as we need, our fear of deprivation vanishes and we experience *habituation*. This means that the more we have of something, the less exciting it becomes. Once you trust that what had been forbidden will never be taken away, you can experience true safety and satisfaction. To make peace with food, you must commit to choosing whatever you feel like eating and in whatever amount satisfies you—forever!*

List all the foods you would like to include in your eating life, including any foods you wish you could eat but have felt you shouldn't. (Feel free to circle back to this list any time and add or cross out foods.)

O ....

O ....

O ....

O ....

O ....

O ....

O ....

O ....

* As a caveat, it is important to state that if you have food scarcity or unreliable access to food, you may not reach that place of habituation out of fear of future deprivation. If so, please have self-compassion for your situation. Habituation will also not take place if you continue to hold thoughts of future diets.

Take a look at the foods you listed in your last entry and choose one that triggers strong feelings of judgment. Write about those judgments. Where did the judgments come from? What do you think it would be like to step away from those judgments and simply allow this food to be in your life, giving you satisfaction? Write it all down.

♥ GO DEEPER: Write a song or a story about a food on your list; draw a cartoon about it or plan a meal around it.

Remember: reconnecting with your inner wisdom is a process, not a straight path. It will be more accessible as you move away from judgments about foods and eating.

Contemplate
other foods you
listed. Where did the
judgments come from? What
would it be like to let go of
them and welcome the
food into your life?

Choose a food that you used to forbid yourself. Choose a time period (a few days or a week) and set an intention to eat as much of it as you like, as often as you like.

What's the food? _____

How many days? _____

What was it like to be allowed to eat it? What feelings did you have? You may have had a lot of different feelings during this practice—write about as many as you can.

GO DEEPER: What would it be like if you made peace with this food permanently? Try it. Notice whether your fear of being out of control or your feelings of deprivation begin to subside. Watch how the food takes its place in your eating life.

Try this with other foods—choose one, invite it in, and see what it's like to have it in your life guilt-free.

Now that you've practiced freeing different foods from rules of diet culture, take this journey out into the world. Set an intention to eat something in a restaurant that you've never freely allowed yourself to choose.

What restaurant will you go to? _____

What will you choose to eat? _____

Notice and write about the feelings you have before you go out, during your time at the restaurant, and after the experience.

_____

_____

_____

_____

_____

_____

_____

_____

_____

_____

_____

_____

_____

_____

_____

_____

_____

_____

Some people describe their immersion in diet culture as living in food jail.

Often, people discover a strange phenomenon that occurs when they've finally broken free from food jail and have made full peace with food: the forbidden foods they once thought were exciting start to lose their thrill. Sometimes people no longer even like them!

Once you've begun to feel some freedom from food jail, go back to the list you made earlier of all of the foods you'd like to have in your eating world. As you look down the list, which foods have you discovered that you truly like? Which have dropped off your desire list because they've lost that thrill?

GO DEEPER: As you've worked to break out of food jail, how is your relationship with food changing? What thoughts and feelings have come up? Or if you like, draw pictures, or write a poem.

CHAPTER 5

Challenge the Food Police

On your journey to reclaiming your inner Intuitive Eater, you may encounter resistance from others in your life. Not everyone has been awakened to the benefits of Intuitive Eating, let alone its principles.

When you hear diet-culture talk from friends or family members, you are experiencing the *External Food Police*. Food Police have bought into weight stigma and the idea that there are "good" and "bad" foods, and they police every bite that goes into their mouths—and, too often, every bite that goes into your mouth. Food Police often have good intentions, but they just end up keeping you in food jail.

Sometimes the food police are real people in your life (including media makers whose work you follow). But often, they are internal voices, including voices from the past that you carry around (mom, coach, college friend, doctor, etc.), or internalized voices that live in your own thought patterns.

In this chapter you'll discover what those voices are saying and practice challenging them so you can have your own, personal, Intuitive Eater voice—the voice that guides you to a new healthy and happy relationship with food and your body.

Recall some of the times and places in your life where you've encountered the Food Police speaking diet culture language, and, if you can, what was said. For example, comments about eliminating certain foods to "benefit your health" or the "obesity epidemic" or "lose weight to get into your bikini".

Where were those voices coming from (for example, social media, magazines, family members, friends, health professionals)? What did they say? Note how old you were, where you were, and who was speaking.

GO DEEPER: Look back at what you just wrote and think about the feelings that arose whenever you got a message from the Food Police.

Several destructive inner voices tend to arise when we're trapped in diet culture. These include:

- *The Internal Food Police:* Acts as your inner judge.
- *The Nutrition Informant:* Gives you "nutrition advice" that colludes with diet culture (rather than supporting your health and wellbeing).
- *The Diet Rebel:* The rebellious teen in you that acts out against diet culture to assert autonomy but is disconnected from your internal wisdom.

Over the next day or two, pay attention to your thoughts about food, eating, and dieting. Which of these voices pervade your thoughts? Do you notice any other destructive or unsupportive voices? What are they saying to you?

You can develop powerful ally inner voices to counter the destructive inner voices and to help you find your *Intuitive Eater* voice. These include:

- *The Food Anthropologist:* Allows you to explore your hunger and fullness signals, your satisfaction levels, and your thoughts and behaviors—WITHOUT judgment.

- *The Rebel Ally:* Helps you protect your private eating and body boundaries from those who try to invade them with diet culture comments.

- *The Nurturer:* Soothes and reassures you with compassion throughout your Intuitive Eating journey.

Over the next day or two, pay careful attention when these voices emerge. Which voice came out? Are there any others you can name? What do they say and how does it help you?

So far in this chapter, you've been getting to know your destructive inner (and outer) voices, as well as your helpful inner voices. Now, you can learn to use your ally voices to counter the Food Police.

You can start by using your ally voices to counter your internal/internalized Food Police.

Here are some examples:

"I am not going to feel guilty if I sometimes miss following my body's hunger or fullness cues."

"I'll treat myself with compassion rather than judgment if I fall into some old thinking."

"I'll notice if I'm feeling rebellious when my internal Food Police try to invade my eating decisions. That feeling will help me fight the inner police voice."

Use one of your rehearsed retorts when you feel your internal food police speak up. Write about what it was like. What did your internal food police say? What did you say back and how did it feel?

Now you can practice using your inner ally voices to help you when dealing with the External Food Police. What are some lines you can use to shut them down?

Here are some examples:

"I've been doing a lot of reading, and I no longer believe that diets work—in fact, they can do a lot of damage to someone's self-esteem."

"Let's talk about something more interesting, like this great movie I just saw."

"Please don't make comments to me about my food or body. Those are in my territory. Thank you."

Now, you try it. Be creative—write whatever you like. No one can judge what you write in your journal!

💜 GO DEEPER: Practice saying these lines. Pretend you're an actor memorizing lines. When the opportunity comes up in the next day or so, use one of your rehearsed lines to counter the External Food Police. Write about what happened. What did the Food Police say? What did you say back and how did it feel?

Certain common thinking patterns reinforce Food Police messages. One is *dichotomous thinking*—or all-or-nothing thinking, which is driven by the need to achieve perfection.

For example:

"I can only eat nutritious foods—no 'junk' food for me." (Note: Intuitive Eaters call foods that are less nutritious "play food," not "junk food.")

"I must exercise every day or not at all. Why bother moving my body, if I can't break a sweat? It's not worth it. I'd rather watch TV."

Over the next day or so, notice and write down any examples of this kind of thinking. Then, alter these thoughts, by thinking in more middle ground terms, instead of all-or-nothing ways, and by using words like "whenever I like" and "sometimes." Notice how that one little change can banish the idea of striving for perfection!

Other thinking patterns that can sabotage your ability to fully embrace Intuitive Eating include:

- *Catastrophic thinking:* Thinking in extremely exaggerated ways, using words like "never" and "always". For example, "If I eat what I want, I'll never stop."

- *Pessimistic thinking:* Feeling hopeless and thinking "the cup is half empty." This makes it difficult to find the joy and pleasure in eating.

- *Linear thinking:* Framing Intuitive Eating as a straight line from beginning to end (as diets do in their focus on weight loss). Be aware of the temptation to turn Intuitive Eating into another diet!

Over the next day or so, notice and write about your thinking patterns. Look at what you wrote and try to counter your thinking in ways that can free you to find your inner Intuitive Eater. For example:

- Use words such as "maybe" or "sometimes".

- Think of how to turn pessimistic thoughts into positive and hopeful thoughts.

- Remind yourself that Intuitive Eating is a flowing process of change with space and time for you to learn and grow.

Read over what you've written in this chapter as you've analyzed your inner eating voices and thinking patterns.

Which of your voices and patterns are most negatively affecting your progress in finding your inner Intuitive Eater voice? Write them here.

Now set an intention to work on changing them. Over the next day or so, practice noticing, countering, and releasing these thoughts. When you do this, what happens? What is it like?

CHAPTER 6

Feel Your Fullness

Intuitive Eating honors the brilliant way our bodies maintain something I call *homeobalance* (rather than homeostasis)—or all the vital physiological processes that keep our bodies going. In just one human cell, there are about a billion chemical reactions every second! Hunger signals remind us that we need food to survive. Fullness signals finish that job by prompting us to eat enough food to meet our body's needs, while not overloading us and making us feel uncomfortable. As an Intuitive Eater, you learn that these signals are accurate and trustworthy.

Besides nourishing ourselves with enough food, eating until we're comfortably full helps us derive the most satisfaction we can from eating. Once you reach comfortable fullness, food just doesn't taste as good as it did when you were hungry and began eating. This chapter will help you hone your fullness awareness so that you can get optimal enjoyment from eating.

Note: it can be difficult to honor, or even notice, fullness if you have food insecurity (a lack of reliable access to enough food) either because of financial limitations or self-imposed restrictions, if you haven't made full peace with food. Making peace with food is a fundamental principle of Intuitive Eating because once you are secure in knowing that you will give yourself a sufficient amount of foods that satisfy your taste buds without judgment or guilt, you will find it less difficult to stop eating when you're comfortably full.

The same chart you used in chapter 3 to look closely at your hunger can be used to find out about your fullness (from 6 to 10).

For the next few days, set an intention to notice which level of fullness you feel at the end of your meals. Make notes about each meal, including what foods you had and your fullness levels afterward. Remember, you're gathering information about your personal experience of fullness outside of any diet culture messages. Just notice what happens at each meal. Use more paper if you run out of room.

FEELINGS OF HUNGER & FULLNESS

Over Hungry	0	Painfully hungry. This is *primal hunger*. It's very intense and can actually hurt.
	1	Ravenous and irritable. An urgent need to eat.
	2	Extremely hungry. Immediate need to find some food.
Comfortable Eating Range	3	Fully hungry and ready to eat.
	4	Mildly hungry, begin noticing hunger.
	5	Neutral. Neither hungry nor full.
	6	Starting to feel satisfied.
	7	Comfortable fullness, feeling completely satisfied and content—a sign to stop.
Over Full	8	Beginning to feel a little too full. Beyond physically needing food.
	9	Extremely full and uncomfortable—everything feels tight.
	10	Stuffed and in pain. Maybe even nauseous.

Continue your exploration by eating normally for another few days, and when you finish, note the fullness level you're at on the fullness scale and, this time, notice the *physical sensations* you experience when you stop eating. For example, you may feel comfortable, satisfied or unsatisfied, or overfull or stuffed. (If you have trouble with this, take a look at the next prompt in this chapter.)

Learning to become attuned to comfortable fullness (about a 7 on the Hunger/Fullness scale) can help you feel better, both physically and emotionally. You'll walk away from your meal feeling satisfied but not uncomfortable.

To reach this goal, practice taking time-outs during your meal to check in with fullness.

Set an intention to check in with your fullness during some meals over the next few days. Notice when you reach the absence of hunger (5), which usually comes after just a few bites but does not indicate fullness. Notice when you begin to feel satisfied but haven't had quite enough (6). Check in with yourself at the midway point, and then again sometime after that. At what point do you reach a 7?

Note: It takes about twenty minutes for your brain to get the message that your stomach is full, so pace your meal accordingly. Please don't judge yourself if you sometimes choose to eat beyond a 7 because the food just tastes so good. This is part of Intuitive Eating. Remember—no rules, no rigidity.

Write about your experience taking time-outs and checking in with your fullness.

♥ GO DEEPER: Notice the emotions you may have connected to your physical sensations of fullness. For example, do you feel calm or happy when you're comfortably full or angry, guilty, or ashamed when you're excessively full? Write about whatever feelings you notice.

If you're having difficulty noticing your physical sensations or emotions while eating, it could be the result of your personal history with dieting and diet culture, childhood experiences, or other environmental factors.

If yo-yo dieting (losing and restoring weight over and over) is part of your history, it may have affected your ability to be in tune with fullness. The survival part of your brain may have lowered your levels of Leptin—a fullness hormone. You may have yo-yo'd between never feeling fullness because you weren't eating enough and habitually eating to over-fullness as you rebounded from deprivation. Write about your experiences.

Were you told to "clean your plate" as a child? If so, you probably have some pretty loud internal policing around that. Try challenging the command to finish everything on your plate by reminding yourself that only you know how much food you need to feel comfortably full. What other counter statements can you come up with? Write them here.

What else might be keeping you from noticing physical sensations of fullness or any emotions that may come up while eating?

Other barriers to noticing fullness include beginning a meal with *primal hunger* (you haven't eaten in multiple hours and you're ravenous) and *distracted eating.*

To avoid getting into primal hunger, notice and write about it when it happens to you. What was the situation (for example, an unexpected emergency or lack of access to food when you started to feel hungry)? Are you chronically overscheduled? How might you protect yourself from that happening again?

The solution to distracted eating, of course, is to take away the distractors that keep you from noticing when you're comfortably full.

List distractors in your life (for example, eating while on the phone, watching TV, surfing the internet, checking your feeds).

Which distractors can you try to remove? What barriers might there be to disconnecting from them?

Have a meal without
distraction. What feelings
come up when you do this?
Did it help you become
more aware of reaching
comfortable fullness?

Remember from chapter 4 the way diet culture makes deprivation and guilt work like a see-saw? The same is true of physical deprivation and over-fullness. Comfortable fullness is the still point at the center of the see-saw, and honoring it means we reject the ups and downs of dieting forever.

If the mere thought of future deprivation (another diet) keeps you filling yourself up past your comfortable capacity, revisit chapter one and try recommitting to stopping dieting forever. Knowing you're committed to your freedom will help you trust your fullness each day.

Then write some affirmations that bring you back to your commitment to embracing Intuitive Eating when you're stuck on the up and down swings of the see-saw.

Some examples:

- I have compassion for myself and my journey.
- I do not listen to the Food Police.
- I trust my body—my hunger and my fullness.
- I give my body what it needs to be satisfied.

Now, write some of your own. Or, if your misgivings have vanished and you're committed to never going on another diet, explore how this is boosting your ability to stop eating when you're comfortably full.

Making peace with all foods goes along with rejecting dieting. If you know that you'll never be forbidden from eating a food you desire, it's easier to talk yourself through stopping eating when you're comfortably full. Tell yourself:

- I'm allowed to eat this food again when I'm hungry again.
- It will be more satisfying to eat it again when I'm hungry than to keep eating it when I'm already full.
- I'll get hungry again today—there are a lot of chances to eat every day.

What else might you say to yourself?

Try this out at your next meal. Write about the feelings that come up when you notice fullness and how it was to talk yourself through them.

Sometimes, a feeling of sadness arises when we stop eating because we're comfortably full. This is called *The Sadness of Saying Enough,* and it's a common feeling when we have to stop doing something enjoyable—whether it's eating a delicious meal, finishing an intriguing book, or coming home from a blissful vacation. It's a feeling that will quickly vanish if you get up from the table and start another activity. (Remember, there are more eating experiences to come!) What are some activities you could have ready, when you're experiencing this sadness? Write about your experience.

CHAPTER 7

Cope with Your Feelings with Kindness

The moment the first taste of milk touches our infant tongues, we learn that eating can be a comforting, satisfying experience—especially if we are fed with consistent and tender care.

Intuitive Eating helps you feed yourself in this same tender way throughout your life. It lets you give yourself permission to enjoy food when you need extra comfort, whether from a special soothing food or more food than you typically eat.

But food can also distract you from your feelings, put you in a numbed state, or even be used as self-punishment. These uses are more likely if food is a primary coping mechanism for you. When food is used for coping, rather than for hunger, nourishment, or joy, eating loses the ability to offer you satisfaction. Be kind to yourself if this is the case. "Emotional eating" can also be a rebound behavior when you feel guilty or ashamed about eating what you like.

In this chapter, you'll explore many ways to cope with emotions once you've made full peace with food. If you need to practice making all foods emotionally equivalent, keep working on the exercises in chapter 4.

Note: If you find yourself frequently eating as a form of escape or self-punishment, consider finding a therapist trained in Intuitive Eating to help you face your deeper feelings.

Set an intention to spend a few days noticing how often you choose to eat in order to deal with an emotional trigger (for example, boredom, sadness, anger, frustration, anxiety, fear, stress, etc.).

Choose one or two of these moments and write about it here. What was the emotional trigger? What was happening that triggered the emotion itself? What foods did you choose to help you cope?

💜 GO DEEPER: Think about how this coping mechanism has worked for you and how it has not. Make a pro/con list to help you explore both the benefits and the drawbacks. (Remember, if you seek food for comfort in trying times, understand that doing so is part of Coping with Your Feelings with Kindness. Food can be a comfort when you really need it! Just remember to stay present while eating, so you can experience the comfort you seek.)

Have you noticed that you frequently seek food to soothe your emotions? If so, when this happens ask yourself the following questions:

1. Am I biologically hungry? (If so, you need to eat.)
2. What am I feeling if not hunger?
3. What do I really need ?
4. What can I ask for to help me get through these feelings?

Write these questions on an index card or put them in a text memo on your phone to remind you to ask them when you are in the moment. You can write down the answers or record a voice memo. Write about any patterns you notice. How can this help you make conscious choices?

Sometimes, when we're young we learn to deny that we have needs (often while taking care of everyone else's needs). This is especially true if our physical and emotional needs are not consistently met by our caregivers.

Here are some basic needs that are often overlooked:

- Getting enough food to nourish ourselves
- Sleeping at least seven to eight hours a night
- Receiving physical touch
- Expressing thoughts and feelings
- Getting emotional support from others
- Pursuing stimulating experiences, both intellectually and creatively

Do you have other core needs that are often overlooked? What are they? Write about one (or more) of your chronically unmet needs.

💜 GO DEEPER: Set an intention to work on getting your basic needs met. What need(s) will you work on? How will you go about it? What challenges do you anticipate? After you've taken some action to meet your needs, reflect and write about how you feel physically and emotionally.

Coping with your feelings with kindness involves both providing nurturance for yourself and finding it from others. Nurturing yourself on a daily basis and asking others for nurturance provides the foundation for being able to handle your difficult feelings.

First, list some ways you can nurture yourself (for example, listening to soothing music, resting and relaxing, meditating, enjoying a good book or film). Now set an intention to try one of these each day for a week. At night, write about what you did and how it felt.

O _____

O _____

O _____

O _____

O _____

O _____

O _____

_____

_____

_____

_____

_____

_____

Now list some ways you can seek nurturance from others (for example, asking for a hug, asking to have your feelings heard, or asking for help).

O _____

O _____

O _____

O _____

O _____

O _____

O _____

Set an intention to ask for one of these needs to be met.

What nurturance will you seek? _____

_____

What challenges might you encounter (for example, fear of rejection or fear of ridicule)? _____

_____

_____

Write about what it was like to seek another's help getting this need met.

_____

_____

When you feel nurtured, you have a better chance of learning to sit with your feelings, rather than trying to escape them. This is called *developing your emotional muscle*. In addition to seeking nurturance from other people, you can practice strengthening your muscle in other ways. Here are some ideas:

- Journal regularly
- Allow yourself to cry when you need to
- Express your feelings through music, art, or physical movement
- Practice affirmations

What other practices might you try to build your emotional muscle?

Write about an experience you've had with sitting with your feelings, rather than escaping them.

💜 GO DEEPER: To practice sitting with a difficult feeling, sit or lie down and mindfully meditate for a few minutes. Pay attention to how your body feels—your feet on the ground, your hands by your side, your back against a chair

- become aware of the sounds around you,
- observe your breathing,
- focus on something in your environment, like a flower or a painting,
- think about someone or some place in your life where you feel safe and comforted,
- now, notice how long you were able to "be" with this feeling without trying to make it go away somehow.

Write about this experience. Is this something you might like to practice regularly, to strengthen your emotional muscle?

Sometimes, it's just too difficult to feel your feelings in the moment. This is often when people distract themselves with food. When you're not able to seek help from a safe person who can nurture you and help you bear your feelings or simply can't sit with your feelings on your own, it can be effective to distract yourself with something other than food. You might read a good book, watch a movie, or start a puzzle.

What else might work for you? Make a list.

Set an intention to try one out the next time you're having difficulty sitting with a feeling.

O _____

O _____

O _____

O _____

O _____

O _____

O _____

If food has been your main coping mechanism throughout your life, it may be the only way you know how to get through difficult times. One important way to help manage life's challenges is to maintain a daily practice of gratitude.

Gratitude can calm your feelings, raise your spirits, and be practiced and built like a muscle.

Start your first gratitude list here by listing the parts of your life for which you are grateful:

- ○
- ○
- ○
- ○
- ○
- ○
- ○
- ○
- ○
- ○
- ○
- ○
- ○

💜 GO DEEPER: Consider starting a separate gratitude journal, try beginning (or ending) each day with a gratitude list. As time goes on, notice how your appreciation for the positive aspects of your life lifts your mood and improves your ability to cope with your difficulties.

CHAPTER 8

Respect Your Body

Every day we are bombarded with diet-culture messages telling us our bodies' size and shape are not acceptable. That we need to "do something" to make our bodies fit the cultural ideal.

Not only do these toxic messages cause us to fear weight-based stigma, but they don't respect that bodies are naturally different. It's absurd to think we could change our height or foot size, yet we are told to spend endless hours trying to change other aspects of our size and shape.

Learning self-hatred from cultural messages, we end up with diminished respect for our bodies. Intuitive Eating teaches us to respect our bodies, inside and out, by learning to ignore those messages and appreciate the gift of life and the body that is our lifelong companion. This chapter will help you practice body respect.

Show respect for your body by nourishing yourself regularly throughout the day. Doing so lets you avoid primal hunger and helps you eat to satisfaction. You have a right to have satisfying meals, whatever else your day contains.

For one or two days, pay attention to the challenges that put you at risk of falling into primal hunger. Do you have a busy day at work ahead? What meals or snacks will you need so that you can begin eating with comfortable hunger and end up with a satisfying experience? What factors could get in the way of this? How can you make sure that you're able to have all the meals you need?

At the end of the day, journal about how your hunger felt throughout the day and whether the meals you ate were satisfying.

Speaking kindly to yourself about your body, and removing any body-bashing statements you've grown accustomed to, can help build deep body respect.

Today, set an intention to stay present, pay attention to how you speak to yourself about your body, and challenge any negative self-talk and replace it with loving self-statements. To get ready, write some positive comments you can use.

Here are some examples:

- I'm grateful that my feet allow me to take a walk in nature.
- I appreciate that my arms can hug someone I love.
- I love the smile on my face when I'm feeling happy.

At the end of the day, write about your experience.

Did you discover any negative body talk? Were you able to throw it out? If not, how did it make you feel? And if you let it go, what were your feelings?

♥ GO DEEPER: Continue to practice replacing or countering negative self-statements with positive ones. As it becomes a habit to use respectful and kind words about your body, reflect on how your feelings about your body have shifted.

We can't respect our bodies if we don't respect body diversity and work to reduce our internal weight bias.

You can begin to reject weight stigma by no longer weighing yourself and by throwing out your scale. Frequent weighing leads you to focus on a number, rather than on your inner characteristics or physical sensations. Trust your body's wisdom rather than the number on the scale.

I first suggested throwing out your scale in chapter 1. If you haven't done it, write about what it might be like to throw out your scale as a gesture of body respect. If you have done it, write about what that has been like for you.

♥ GO DEEPER: Set an intention to notice any internal weight bias you carry toward others. What would it feel like to respect body diversity in others? How can it help you be kinder to yourself and more accepting of your own body, regardless of its size or shape? Write about your thoughts and feelings.

When you dress in comfortable ways that honor your style preferences, it shows kindness and respect for your body.

Set aside a few hours and throw out or donate clothes that don't fit your here-and-now body. (If you can afford it, buy a few new pieces of clothing that fit you well and that you can enjoy wearing.)

This process might bring up some deep feelings. Write about your thoughts and feelings about only keeping clothes that fit your body just as it is.

Comparing your body to others is disrespectful to your body. It dishonors your true essence. It reinforces feelings of envy of others and dissatisfaction with yourself, leading to deep unhappiness.

What would it be like to commit to eliminating these behaviors? What challenges might you face? What actions could you take to start leaving body comparisons behind?

Your body is far more than its size or shape. Thinking about everything your body does every day can help you build gratitude for how it functions and the miracle of how it has gotten you through life. Write about some of the many amazing things your body does (like your heart constantly beating and your lungs regularly breathing).

💜 GO DEEPER: Think deeply about the inner aspects of yourself that you can appreciate and admire—consider your personality, intelligence, wit, listening capacity, and values; how you treat others; and more. List your inner qualities here (use all the extra paper you need!):

What else can you do to show respect for your physical body? Think about:

- Ways you can pamper yourself
- Ways you can receive the touch that your body needs
- Ways you can get better sleep

Write your ideas here. Perhaps you could get a massage, a loving hug from someone safe, or take a nap. What else?

If you set an intention to give your body these loving gifts, do you anticipate any difficulties or challenges fulfilling this intention? How might you overcome these challenges?

O

O

O

O

O

O

O

O

O

O

O

O

💜 GO DEEPER: Another way to show respect for your body is to move in pleasurable ways. Moving your body raises "feel-good" hormones, offers you more physical ease, and creates new neural pathways that support mental and emotional wellbeing. What do you do each day to move your body in ways you enjoy? What would you like to do more? (You will explore this more in the next chapter.)

Review the prompts in this chapter, and ask yourself which aspects of showing respect for your body might deserve more attention? Which resonate most with you? As you practice respecting your body, do you notice that your relationship with your body begins to relax and that you're able to be more accepting of body diversity—both yours and others?

Write about your progress toward respecting your body and how that feels, both physically and emotionally.

CHAPTER 9

Movement—
Feel the Difference

Whether it's a wriggling baby in your arms, a toddler struggling with their first steps, or children running around the playground—people are meant to move.

Yet cultural messages tell us that unless we're sweating at a gym or running a marathon, we aren't moving our bodies right.

Nothing could be farther from the truth. As creatures built to move, any movement is good for us: walking, dancing, stretching, bending down to pull weeds, carrying shopping bags into the house. It's all good for us in a myriad of ways. Frequent movement can give us increased flexibility, strength, balance, stamina, and agility. It can improve our heart function, bone density, immune system functioning, and sleep. It can also reduce stress and calm nerves.

This chapter is about exploring your relationship with movement and the ways that movement can give you a better quality of life.

There's an acronym that describes the benefits of movement: NEAT (non-exercise activity thermogenesis).

NEAT describes the energy burned by any kind of movement you do throughout the day that's not formal exercise. Walking up and down stairs, cleaning your house, taking walks along the beach, gardening, dancing—all of these have huge positive impacts on our physical and mental health.

How might you bring more NEAT into your life? If it feels overwhelming, start by considering all the baby steps (literally and figurately) you can take.

For example, stretch your arms and legs before you get out of bed in the morning. If you're on the computer all day, take a few minutes each hour to stand up and walk around, or make a few dance moves while you're getting dressed in the morning. Which tiny, baby steps will you take?

Once you've begun to see how much NEAT you can incorporate through baby steps, you can begin to bring even more NEAT into your life. This starts with motivation, but sometimes there are real obstacles in our lives that make it difficult to make changes.

What obstacles to moving more exist in your life (for example, illness, weather, time constraints, or lack of space for indoor exercise equipment)? What are yours?

What are your thoughts or feelings about these obstacles?

GO DEEPER: Think about ways to challenge these obstacles. Do you feel you don't have time for movement? Maybe you can set an intention to use five minutes of your lunch break to walk outside. If you don't have someone to watch your kids while you exercise, involve them: toss a ball or walk the dog together. If you have a disability, do you have safe and welcome support for and access to movement with any modifications you might need? Write your ideas here and make an intention to try some of them.

Are you resistant to exercise? Sometimes people develop difficult feelings about exercise when they equate it with weight loss, have an injury, feel physically inadequate, or were pushed to exercise as a child.

In your life, have you embraced exercise/movement, or have you been resistant to including it in your life? What is your history with exercise? Write about any exercise resistance you may have.

Many diet culture messages promote exercise as a way to lose weight. If you have believed these messages during times you have dieted, they may be deeply entrenched, and it may be difficult to shift your attitude toward movement. Write about the impact that diet culture still has on you. Perhaps, re-read what you wrote in chapter 1 to get started.

What ways can you think of to disconnect the ideas of exercise and weight loss? How might you embrace movement as a way to FEEL better, rather than to look a certain way or see a certain number on the scale?

What is your idea of pleasurable movement—movement that can bring joy into your life? Maybe you like dancing, playing a sport, stretching and strengthening your muscles with yoga, swimming in the ocean or a lake, taking a long walk with a friend. Draw a picture of yourself moving in a way that feels good or describe it with words.

If you've begun to move on a regular basis, notice any changes in your belief system, emotions, or physical and mental well-being.

Write about these changes.

When we are compulsively caught up in exercise (rather than movement), we're apt to ignore signs from our bodies that we're over-doing it—maybe a pulled muscle, a cold coming on, or simple exhaustion. Incorporating pleasurable movement means listening to all the messages your body gives you—and this means embracing the need to regularly rest your body, especially when it "speaks up".

Do you give yourself the gift of rest? If not, examine your thoughts about the purpose of movement in your life. What intention can you set to be kinder to your body when it signals you that it needs to take a break from movement?

CHAPTER 10

Honor Your Health with Gentle Nutrition

There is great intention and purpose in leaving nutrition for the very end of the journey toward Intuitive Eating.

Before you can engage with nutrition, you need to:

- challenge (and banish) diet culture messages.
- decide that satisfaction is a priority in your eating life.
- make full peace with food.
- find kind ways of coping with your emotions.
- learn to be respectful to your body.

When you have fully embraced these principles, you may begin to listen to how your body feels in relation to food and eating. In this chapter, you will begin to explore how nutrition can boost your physical well-being.

Before you start, consider whether you've made all foods emotionally equivalent, meaning you don't feel good or bad based on your food choice. As you work through this chapter, if anything begins to trigger an old desire to judge the foods you choose, you may not yet be ready to explore nutrition. That's okay. Consider rereading chapter 4 on making peace with food. It takes some people longer than others to explore how their nutrition interacts with their health and energy. You'll get there!

Let's begin with the concept of "playfood". We often label foods we think are forbidden as "junk-food." But "junk" implies something to throw out, while "play" is something we need in our lives on a regular basis. So playfood is food that may have limited nutritional value but is definitely one of the pleasures of life.

To explore playfood, take notice of your intuitive eating for about a week. Take pictures of a few meals, write about them, or simply put them in your memory bank.

At the end of the week, take a little time to think about your meals. Have you naturally desired and eaten a variety of foods? Write about your experience with both foods that you think are filled with nutrients and foods that are simply there for delight.

Put your focus on how you feel physically. Over the next week, notice:

- your energy level throughout each day.
- the functioning of your gastrointestinal tract. Any stomach aches, constipation, gas, or bloating?
- any headaches, brain fog, sleepiness, or low energy?

DAY ONE

DAY TWO

DAY THREE

DAY FOUR

DAY FIVE

DAY SIX

DAY SEVEN

All of the physical sensations you experience are examples of your body giving you messages. The awareness of messages that come from within is called *interoceptive awareness*.

Now, let's explore the links between nutrition and body messages—energy levels, digestive function, headaches and sleepiness.

What messages are you getting, pleasant or unpleasant or somewhere in between? Just notice without judging, learning more and more about your body's relationship to the foods you take into it.

This week, pay attention to your energy levels. Take note each day of when your energy ebbs and flows.

Is your energy pretty uneven? It might be that the *frequency* and *balance* of your meals could be adjusted. In other words, eating more often and including a balance of carbohydrate, protein, and fat in most meals may even out your energy.

Try adding more complex carbs to your meals (oatmeal, starchy veggies, whole wheat bread, and so on). And if your meals tend to be low on protein or fat, add some cheese or peanut butter or fish (for example) to even out your blood sugar.

If you find that you often get really hungry and experience low-energy between meals, try having four or five smaller meals, regularly spaced, instead of three. Different mealtimes work for different people.

Experiment with balance and frequency until you're feeling more consistent energy throughout the day. What works for you?

DAY ONE

DAY TWO

DAY THREE

DAY FOUR

DAY FIVE

DAY SIX

DAY SEVEN

Are you experiencing constipation? It's possible that you could use more fiber in your meals. Whole grains, beans, nuts, fruits, and vegetables offer great sources of fiber. Try adding more of these high-fiber foods for a few days and see if the change helps relieve the constipation. Also, be sure to drink plenty of water. How does it feel physically to pay attention to adding these foods?

How does it feel, emotionally, to keep these changes in mind?

If you're having any GI distress (gas, stomach aches, bloating), there are a few ways that diet might be contributing. It's possible you have a lactose intolerance when you eat a dairy food, which means that your body can't break down the molecules in lactose, so it ferments causing gas and bloating. Also, certain vegetables, such as cauliflower, Brussel sprouts, or broccoli, cause gas in some people. Beans can do that too.

For a week, pay attention to how your GI distress tracks with dairy, cruciferous veggies, or beans. Write what you notice.

If you find links, this doesn't mean you have to cut foods you love out of your diet. Try varying the amount you eat of foods you think are making you physically uncomfortable to help sort out how much you can eat without excessive distress. You might also want to try a digestive enzyme, like Beano. For dairy, taking one or more lactase tablets can help, with the first bite of anything that contains dairy.

Write about what you've discovered. Are there any changes you can make to feel better? What choices work best for you?

If you experience headaches or sleepiness, there are a few ways your intake might be affecting you. If you wait too long to eat, or suddenly decrease the amount of caffeine you're taking in, you may end up with a headache. (Avoid stopping your caffeine intake cold turkey. If you want to decrease, do it gradually!)

If you eat a meal that's mostly carbohydrate, this can raise your serotonin levels and make you sleepy. Maybe have the pasta at dinner, rather than lunch, if you have this reaction. Or add protein to your meal to keep you more alert.

If you have noticed that your eating choices are linked to sleepiness or headaches, write about it here. What changes, if any, will work best for you? Remember, you are free to make any choice you want: sometimes the tradeoff is worth it. You get to decide.

Our media world is full of food fads that promise you miraculous changes in the size of your body or how your body feels. They promise you quick results and may be recommended by famous people. Some urge you to eliminate certain foods or food groups—like cutting out sugar or even most carbohydrates. Some tout certain supplements or "magic" foods like apple cider vinegar, or ways of eating, like "clean eating". Although there isn't reliable scientific evidence to support them, sometimes it feels like they really work—for a while. The power of suggestion can be very strong. Believing that some food will make us feel better or worse can actually impact how we feel. That's called the placebo or nocebo effect—and it's part of the mind-body connection.

Unfortunately, some very uncomfortable or even dangerous effects can result from these fad diets like fatigue, gastrointestinal problems, or headaches. And even if this doesn't happen, it's difficult to keep up these restricted ways of eating. Just like any diet, they can leave you feeling like a failure.

Have you experienced any of these fads? Write about your experience with them.

💜 GO DEEPER: Review all the observations you have made about how your body responds to the foods you eat and the way you eat. What do you notice? Are you ready to bring gentle nutrition into your life, or do you need more time to practice some of the other Intuitive Eating principles? Not only can gentle nutrition increase your sense of well-being, but being kind with yourself as you find your inner Intuitive Eater, will put you on the path of self-acceptance and joy and pleasure in eating.

YOUR INTUITIVE EATING TOOLBOX

Now that you've gone through all of the prompts in this journal and taken time to explore your thoughts and feelings, sit back with the joy that comes with knowing your inner Intuitive Eater.

Any time you are tempted by the toxic world of diet culture, you can return to this journal to remember why you've decided to let that go and trust your inner wisdom.

List the top three most powerful journal pages that have helped you on your Intuitive Eating journey.

1. _____

2. _____

3. _____

Which prompts helped you the most to:

Get more satisfaction in your eating _____

_____

_____

_____

Notice the different signs of hunger _____

_____

_____

_____

Help you deal with difficult feelings

Appreciate what your body can do and have more body respect

Speak up about your convictions around fighting diet culture

Revisit these prompts when you want to reconnect with a practice or a concept that's been helpful for you.

In short, your journal is a toolbox containing all the tools you need to free your thoughts from diet culture, challenge negative feelings that arise, and practice the behaviors that a committed Intuitive Eater exhibits in their relationship with food and their body.

Keep your journal handy so it's there for you whenever you need it.

MORE WAYS TO HARNESS
THE POWER OF INTUITIVE EATING

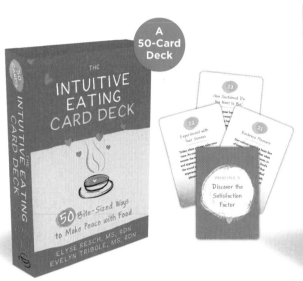

A 50-Card Deck

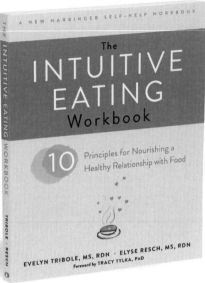

The Intuitive Eating Card Deck
50 Bite-Sized Ways to Make
Peace with Food
978-1684038282 / US $17.95

The Intuitive Eating Workbook
10 Principles for Nourishing a
Healthy Relationship with Food
978-1626256224 / US $24.95

ABOUT THE AUTHOR

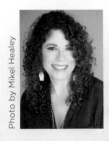

Photo by Mikel Healey

Elyse Resch, MS, RDN, is a nutrition therapist in private practice in Beverly Hills, CA; with more than thirty-nine years of experience specializing in eating disorders, Intuitive Eating, and Health at Every Size. She is author of *The Intuitive Eating Workbook for Teens*, coauthor of *Intuitive Eating* and *The Intuitive Eating Workbook*, and chapter contributor to *Handbook of Positive Body Image and Embodiment*. She is a fellow of the Academy of Nutrition and Dietetics, a certified eating disorder registered dietitian (CEDRD-S), a fellow of the International Association of Eating Disorders Professionals, and supervises and trains dietitians, psychotherapists, and other health professionals.